HASHIMOTO PLANT-BASED COOKBOOK

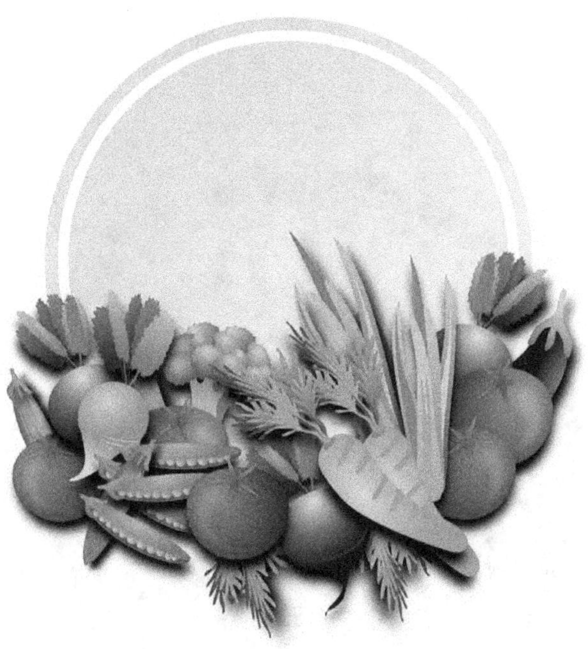

DR. VICKIE STOCK

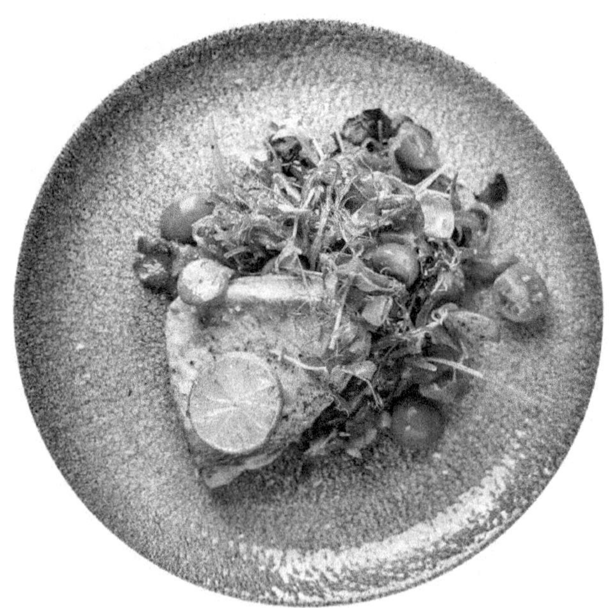

TABLE OF CONTENT

CHAPTER ONE

Understanding Hashimoto's Disease

Hashimoto's disease, also known as Hashimoto's thyroiditis, is an autoimmune condition that affects the thyroid gland, a small butterfly-shaped gland located in the front of the neck.

Named after the Japanese physician Dr. Hakaru Hashimoto, who first described it in 1912, Hashimoto's disease is the most common cause of hypothyroidism in the United States and other developed countries.

Pathophysiology:

Hashimoto's disease occurs when the body's immune system mistakenly attacks the thyroid gland, leading to inflammation and gradual destruction of thyroid tissue.

This autoimmune response disrupts the thyroid's ability to produce thyroid hormones, namely thyroxine (T4) and triiodothyronine (T3), which regulate metabolism, energy levels, body temperature, and other vital functions. As thyroid tissue is damaged, hormone levels decrease, resulting in hypothyroidism.

Risk Factors:

While the exact cause of Hashimoto's disease is not fully understood, several factors may contribute to its development:

Genetics: Individuals with a family history of autoimmune diseases, including Hashimoto's disease, have a higher risk of developing the condition.

Gender: Hashimoto's disease is more common in women than men, with women being diagnosed at a ratio of 10 to 1 compared to men.

Age: While Hashimoto's disease can occur at any age, it is most commonly diagnosed in middle-aged women.

Environmental Triggers: Certain environmental factors, such as exposure to radiation, iodine intake, viral infections, and stress, may trigger or exacerbate autoimmune responses in susceptible individuals.

Symptoms:

Hashimoto's disease often progresses slowly over time, and symptoms may be subtle or nonspecific, making it challenging to diagnose. Common symptoms of Hashimoto's disease include:

- ❖ Fatigue
- ❖ Weight gain
- ❖ Cold intolerance
- ❖ Constipation
- ❖ Dry skin
- ❖ Hair thinning or loss
- ❖ Joint pain

❖ Muscle weakness

❖ Depression

❖ Memory problems

❖ Menstrual irregularities

❖ Diagnosis:

Diagnosing Hashimoto's disease typically involves a combination of medical history, physical examination, and laboratory tests. Key diagnostic tests include:

❖ Thyroid Function Tests: Blood tests measure levels of thyroid-stimulating hormone (TSH), free thyroxine (T4), and triiodothyronine (T3). In Hashimoto's disease, TSH levels are elevated, while T4 levels are often decreased.

❖ Thyroid Antibody Tests: Blood tests detect the presence of antibodies against thyroid peroxidase (TPO antibodies) and thyroglobulin (TG antibodies), which are indicative of autoimmune thyroiditis.

❖ Ultrasound Imaging: Thyroid ultrasound may reveal characteristic features of Hashimoto's disease, such as a diffusely enlarged thyroid gland with a heterogeneous echotexture.

Treatment:

While Hashimoto's disease is a chronic condition with no cure, it can be effectively managed with lifelong treatment aimed at restoring thyroid hormone levels and alleviating symptoms. Treatment options include:

- ❖ Thyroid Hormone Replacement Therapy: The mainstay of treatment involves taking synthetic thyroid hormone medication, such as levothyroxine (Synthroid), to replace deficient thyroid hormone levels.
- ❖ Regular Monitoring: Patients with Hashimoto's disease require regular monitoring of thyroid function through blood tests to ensure optimal hormone levels and adjust medication dosage as needed.
- ❖ Healthy Lifestyle Practices: Adopting a healthy lifestyle, including a balanced diet, regular exercise, stress management techniques, and adequate sleep, can support overall well-being and thyroid health.
- ❖ Avoiding Iodine Excess: Some individuals with Hashimoto's disease may benefit from avoiding excessive iodine intake, as high iodine levels can exacerbate thyroid inflammation and hormone imbalances.
- ❖ Managing Comorbidities: Hashimoto's disease may increase the risk of other autoimmune conditions, such as celiac disease, type 1 diabetes, and rheumatoid arthritis. Managing these comorbidities through appropriate treatment and lifestyle modifications is essential.

Benefits of a Plant-Based Diet for Hashimoto's Disease

Hashimoto's disease is an autoimmune condition that affects the thyroid gland, leading to inflammation, impaired thyroid function, and symptoms of hypothyroidism.

While medical treatment with thyroid hormone replacement therapy is the primary approach to managing Hashimoto's disease, adopting a plant-based diet can offer additional benefits for individuals with this condition.

A plant-based diet focuses on consuming whole, minimally processed foods derived from plants, such as fruits, vegetables, grains, legumes, nuts, and seeds, while minimizing or avoiding animal products and processed foods. Here are some of the potential benefits of a plant-based diet for individuals with Hashimoto's disease:

1. Reduced Inflammation:

Plant-based diets are rich in antioxidants, phytonutrients, and anti-inflammatory compounds that can help reduce inflammation throughout the body, including in the thyroid gland. Chronic inflammation is a hallmark of autoimmune diseases like Hashimoto's disease, and adopting a diet that helps quell inflammation may help alleviate symptoms and slow disease progression.

2. Improved Gut Health:

The health of the gut microbiota plays a crucial role in regulating the immune system and modulating inflammation. Plant-based diets are high in fiber, which serves as fuel for beneficial gut bacteria.

By promoting a diverse and balanced gut microbiome, a plant-based diet may support immune function and reduce the risk of autoimmune flare-ups in individuals with Hashimoto's disease.

3. Hormone Balance:

Whole plant foods are naturally low in saturated fat and cholesterol and contain phytoestrogens, which are plant-based compounds that can help modulate estrogen levels in the body.

Hormonal imbalances, including disruptions in estrogen metabolism, may contribute to thyroid dysfunction in some individuals. A plant-based diet may help promote hormonal balance and support thyroid health.

4. Weight Management:

Excess weight and obesity are risk factors for Hashimoto's disease and may exacerbate symptoms such as fatigue and joint pain. Plant-based diets tend to be lower in calories and saturated fat while higher in fiber and nutrient density compared to omnivorous diets. By emphasizing whole, nutrient-rich foods and minimizing processed and high-calorie foods, a plant-based diet can support weight management and improve metabolic health.

5. Nutrient Density:

Plant-based diets are abundant in vitamins, minerals, antioxidants, and other micronutrients essential for thyroid function and overall health. Foods such as leafy greens, cruciferous vegetables, berries, nuts, seeds, and whole grains provide an array of nutrients that support immune function, metabolism, energy production, and cellular repair—all of which are important for individuals with Hashimoto's disease.

6. Heart Health:

Individuals with Hashimoto's disease are at an increased risk of cardiovascular disease, partly due to the effects of hypothyroidism on lipid metabolism. Plant-based diets have been associated with lower blood pressure, improved cholesterol levels, and reduced risk of heart disease.

By promoting heart health through a diet rich in fruits, vegetables, whole grains, and healthy fats, individuals with Hashimoto's disease can mitigate cardiovascular risk factors and improve overall well-being.

7. Sustainable Eating:

In addition to the health benefits, adopting a plant-based diet aligns with principles of sustainability and environmental stewardship. Plant-based diets have a lower environmental footprint compared to diets high in animal products, as they require fewer natural resources, produce fewer greenhouse gas emissions, and minimize animal welfare concerns. Choosing plant-based foods can contribute to a more sustainable food system and support environmental conservation efforts.

How to Use this cookbook

Adopting a plant-based diet can offer numerous benefits for individuals with Hashimoto's disease, including reduced inflammation, improved gut health, hormone balance, weight management, nutrient density, heart health, and sustainability.

By prioritizing whole, minimally processed plant foods and minimizing or avoiding animal products and processed foods, individuals with Hashimoto's disease can support their immune system, optimize thyroid function, and enhance overall health and well-being.

While a plant-based diet may not cure Hashimoto's disease, it can complement medical treatment and lifestyle modifications to help individuals manage their condition effectively and improve their quality of life.

As with any dietary change, it's essential to work with a healthcare professional or registered dietitian to ensure nutritional adequacy and personalized support.

Understanding Hashimoto's Disease: Begin by reading the introductory section, which provides essential information about Hashimoto's disease, including its causes, symptoms, diagnosis, and treatment options. Understanding the underlying mechanisms of the condition can empower you to make informed dietary choices.

Benefits of a Plant-Based Diet: Delve into the chapter that explores the benefits of a plant-based diet for Hashimoto's disease in detail. Learn about how plant-based foods can reduce inflammation, support gut health, optimize thyroid function, and promote overall well-being.

Recipe Selection: Explore the diverse range of plant-based recipes tailored specifically for individuals with Hashimoto's disease. The recipes are categorized into different meal types, including breakfast, lunch, dinner, snacks, and desserts, making it easy to plan balanced and nutritious meals throughout the day.

Meal Planning and Preparation: Use the recipes provided in this cookbook as a foundation for meal planning.

Consider your personal preferences, dietary restrictions, and nutritional needs when selecting recipes. Plan your meals for the week ahead, considering factors such as variety, balance, and convenience.

Ingredient Substitutions: Feel free to customize the recipes based on your preferences and ingredient availability. Substitute ingredients as needed, and experiment with different flavor combinations to suit your taste preferences. Consider consulting with a healthcare professional or registered dietitian for personalized dietary advice.

Cooking Instructions: Follow the detailed cooking instructions provided for each recipe. Pay attention to cooking techniques, portion sizes, and serving suggestions to ensure optimal results. Don't hesitate to adjust seasoning, cooking times, or methods to suit your taste and dietary preferences.

Portion Control and Moderation: While plant-based foods are nutritious, portion control is still important, especially for individuals managing Hashimoto's disease. Be mindful of portion sizes and aim for balanced meals that include a variety of nutrient-dense foods.

Enjoyment and Experimentation: Embrace the journey of discovering new flavors and textures as you explore plant-based cooking.

Use this cookbook as a tool for culinary creativity and experimentation, and don't forget to savor the delicious and nourishing meals you create.

Seek Support and Guidance: Remember that dietary changes can be challenging, and it's essential to seek support from loved ones, healthcare professionals, or online communities. Share your experiences, ask questions, and seek guidance as needed to ensure success on your plant-based journey.

CHAPTER TWO

Plant-based Hashimoto Recipes

1: Green Smoothie Bowl

Ingredients:

- ❖ 1 ripe banana
- ❖ 1 cup spinach leaves
- ❖ 1/2 cup frozen mango chunks
- ❖ 1/2 cup unsweetened almond milk
- ❖ 1 tablespoon chia seeds
- ❖ Toppings: sliced strawberries, blueberries, granola, shredded coconut

Instructions:

- ❖ In a blender, combine banana, spinach, mango chunks, almond milk, and chia seeds.
- ❖ Blend until smooth and creamy.
- ❖ Pour the smoothie into a bowl.
- ❖ Top with sliced strawberries, blueberries, granola, and shredded coconut.
- ❖ Enjoy immediately.

Health Benefits:

- Spinach is rich in vitamins and minerals, including iron and vitamin C, which support thyroid health.
- Chia seeds provide omega-3 fatty acids and fiber, which help regulate blood sugar levels and support digestive health.

Preparation Time: 5 minutes

2: Avocado Toast with Tomato and Hemp Seeds

Ingredients:

- 2 slices whole grain bread, toasted
- 1 ripe avocado, mashed
- 1 medium tomato, sliced
- 2 tablespoons hemp seeds
- Pinch of red pepper flakes (optional)
- Pinch of sea salt

Instructions:

- Spread mashed avocado evenly onto each slice of toasted bread.
- Top with sliced tomato.
- Sprinkle hemp seeds over the tomato slices.
- Add a pinch of red pepper flakes and sea salt for extra flavor, if desired.
- Serve immediately.

Health Benefits:

- ❖ Avocado provides healthy fats and potassium, which are beneficial for heart health and may help reduce inflammation.
- ❖ Hemp seeds are a good source of plant-based protein and omega-3 fatty acids, which support brain function and reduce inflammation.

Preparation Time: 10 minutes

3: Quinoa Breakfast Bowl

Ingredients:

- ❖ 1/2 cup cooked quinoa
- ❖ 1/2 cup unsweetened almond milk
- ❖ 1 tablespoon maple syrup
- ❖ 1/2 teaspoon ground cinnamon
- ❖ 1/2 ripe banana, sliced
- ❖ 1/4 cup fresh berries (such as raspberries or blueberries)
- ❖ 1 tablespoon chopped nuts (such as almonds or walnuts)
- ❖ Drizzle of almond butter (optional)

Instructions:

- ❖ In a small saucepan, heat the cooked quinoa with almond milk, maple syrup, and ground cinnamon until warmed through.

❖ Transfer the quinoa mixture to a bowl.

❖ Top with sliced banana, fresh berries, and chopped nuts.

❖ Drizzle with almond butter, if desired.

❖ Serve warm and enjoy!

Health Benefits:

❖ Quinoa is a gluten-free whole grain that provides protein, fiber, and essential amino acids.

❖ Berries are rich in antioxidants and vitamins, which help reduce inflammation and support immune health.

Preparation Time: 10 minutes

4: Sweet Potato Breakfast Hash

Ingredients:

❖ 1 large sweet potato, peeled and diced

❖ 1 tablespoon olive oil

❖ 1/2 small onion, diced

❖ 1 bell pepper, diced

❖ 1 cup baby spinach leaves

❖ 1/2 teaspoon paprika

❖ Salt and pepper to taste

❖ Fresh parsley for garnish (optional)

Instructions:

- ❖ Heat olive oil in a skillet over medium heat.
- ❖ Add diced sweet potato to the skillet and cook until tender, about 8-10 minutes.
- ❖ Add diced onion and bell pepper to the skillet and cook until softened, about 5 minutes.
- ❖ Stir in baby spinach leaves and cook until wilted, about 2 minutes.
- ❖ Season with paprika, salt, and pepper.
- ❖ Garnish with fresh parsley, if desired.
- ❖ Serve hot and enjoy!

Health Benefits:

- ❖ Sweet potatoes are rich in beta-carotene, which is converted to vitamin A in the body and supports immune function.
- ❖ Spinach is a nutrient-dense leafy green vegetable that provides vitamins and minerals, including iron and folate, which are important for thyroid health.

Preparation Time: 20 minutes

5: Berry Chia Seed Pudding

Ingredients:

- ❖ 1/4 cup chia seeds
- ❖ 1 cup unsweetened almond milk

- ❖ 1 tablespoon maple syrup or honey (optional)
- ❖ 1/2 teaspoon vanilla extract
- ❖ 1/2 cup mixed berries (such as strawberries, blueberries, raspberries)
- ❖ 2 tablespoons sliced almonds or chopped walnuts

Instructions:

- ❖ In a bowl, whisk together chia seeds, almond milk, maple syrup or honey (if using), and vanilla extract.
- ❖ Let the mixture sit for 10 minutes, then whisk again to break up any clumps.
- ❖ Cover and refrigerate overnight or for at least 4 hours until the chia seeds have absorbed the liquid and the mixture has thickened.
- ❖ To serve, divide the chia seed pudding into bowls and top with mixed berries and sliced almonds or chopped walnuts.
- ❖ Enjoy chilled!

Health Benefits:

- ❖ Chia seeds are rich in fiber and omega-3 fatty acids, which help regulate blood sugar levels and support heart health.
- ❖ Berries are packed with antioxidants and vitamins, which help reduce inflammation and support immune function.

Preparation Time: 5 minutes (plus chilling time)

Ingredients:

- ❖ 1 tablespoon olive oil
- ❖ 1/2 block (7 oz) firm tofu, crumbled
- ❖ 1/4 teaspoon turmeric powder
- ❖ 1/4 teaspoon garlic powder
- ❖ 1/4 teaspoon onion powder
- ❖ 1/4 teaspoon paprika
- ❖ Salt and pepper to taste
- ❖ 1 cup chopped vegetables (such as bell peppers, onions, spinach)
- ❖ 2 slices whole grain bread, toasted (optional)

Instructions:

- ❖ Heat olive oil in a skillet over medium heat.
- ❖ Add crumbled tofu to the skillet and season with turmeric powder, garlic powder, onion powder, paprika, salt, and pepper.
- ❖ Cook for 5-7 minutes, stirring occasionally, until the tofu is heated through and lightly golden.
- ❖ Add chopped vegetables to the skillet and cook for an additional 3-5 minutes, until the vegetables are tender.
- ❖ Serve the tofu scramble hot, with toasted whole grain bread if desired.

❖ Enjoy!

Health Benefits:

❖ Tofu is a good source of plant-based protein and contains all nine essential amino acids, making it a nutritious alternative to eggs.

❖ Vegetables add vitamins, minerals, and antioxidants to the dish, supporting overall health and well-being.

Preparation Time: 15 minutes

7: Oatmeal with Almond Butter and Banana

Ingredients:

❖ 1/2 cup rolled oats

❖ 1 cup unsweetened almond milk

❖ 1 ripe banana, mashed

❖ 1 tablespoon almond butter

❖ 1 tablespoon maple syrup or honey (optional)

❖ Pinch of cinnamon

❖ Sliced banana and chopped almonds for topping

Instructions:

❖ In a saucepan, combine rolled oats and almond milk. Bring to a boil, then reduce heat and simmer for 5-7 minutes, stirring occasionally, until oats are cooked and mixture has thickened.

- ❖ Stir in mashed banana, almond butter, maple syrup or honey (if using), and cinnamon until well combined.
- ❖ Remove from heat and transfer oatmeal to a bowl.
- ❖ Top with sliced banana and chopped almonds.
- ❖ Serve hot and enjoy!

Health Benefits:

- ❖ Oats are a good source of soluble fiber, which helps regulate blood sugar levels and support digestive health.
- ❖ Almond butter provides healthy fats and protein, which help keep you feeling full and satisfied.

Preparation Time: 10 minutes

8: Coconut Yogurt Parfait

Ingredients:

- ❖ 1 cup unsweetened coconut yogurt
- ❖ 1/2 cup mixed berries (such as strawberries, blueberries, raspberries)
- ❖ 1/4 cup granola (look for a low-sugar or homemade option)
- ❖ 1 tablespoon shredded coconut
- ❖ Drizzle of honey or maple syrup (optional)

Instructions:

- ❖ In a glass or bowl, layer coconut yogurt, mixed berries, and granola.
- ❖ Repeat layers until ingredients are used up.
- ❖ Sprinkle shredded coconut on top.
- ❖ Drizzle with honey or maple syrup if desired.
- ❖ Serve immediately and enjoy!

Health Benefits:

- ❖ Coconut yogurt is dairy-free and rich in probiotics, which support gut health and immune function.
- ❖ Berries are packed with antioxidants and vitamins, which help reduce inflammation and support overall health.

Preparation Time: 5 minutes

9: Chickpea Flour Pancakes

Ingredients:

- ❖ 1 cup chickpea flour
- ❖ 1 tablespoon ground flaxseed
- ❖ 1 teaspoon baking powder
- ❖ 1/2 teaspoon ground cinnamon
- ❖ Pinch of salt
- ❖ 3/4 cup unsweetened almond milk
- ❖ 1 tablespoon maple syrup

- ❖ 1 teaspoon vanilla extract

- ❖ Coconut oil or cooking spray for greasing the pan

- ❖ Fresh fruit for topping (such as sliced bananas or berries)

Instructions:

- ❖ In a mixing bowl, whisk together chickpea flour, ground flaxseed, baking powder, cinnamon, and salt.

- ❖ In a separate bowl, combine almond milk, maple syrup, and vanilla extract.

- ❖ Pour the wet ingredients into the dry ingredients and mix until smooth.

- ❖ Heat a non-stick skillet or griddle over medium heat and lightly grease with coconut oil or cooking spray.

- ❖ Pour about 1/4 cup of batter onto the skillet for each pancake.

- ❖ Cook for 2-3 minutes on each side, until golden brown and cooked through.

- ❖ Serve hot with fresh fruit toppings and a drizzle of maple syrup.

Health Benefits:

- ❖ Chickpea flour is high in protein and fiber, which help stabilize blood sugar levels and promote digestive health.

- ❖ Ground flaxseed provides omega-3 fatty acids and lignans, which have anti-inflammatory properties.

Preparation Time: 15 minutes

10: Veggie Breakfast Burrito

Ingredients:

- ❖ 1 whole grain or sprouted grain tortilla
- ❖ 1/2 cup cooked quinoa
- ❖ 1/4 cup black beans, drained and rinsed
- ❖ 2 tablespoons salsa
- ❖ 1/4 avocado, sliced
- ❖ Handful of baby spinach leaves
- ❖ Sliced bell peppers and onions (optional)
- ❖ Sliced jalapenos (optional)
- ❖ Fresh cilantro for garnish (optional)

Instructions:

- ❖ Lay the tortilla flat on a plate or cutting board.
- ❖ Spread cooked quinoa in the center of the tortilla.
- ❖ Top with black beans, salsa, avocado slices, baby spinach leaves, and any additional vegetables or toppings of your choice.
- ❖ Fold in the sides of the tortilla, then roll it up tightly from the bottom to form a burrito.
- ❖ Heat a skillet over medium heat and lightly toast the burrito on all sides until golden brown and crispy.

❖ Serve hot, garnished with fresh cilantro if desired.

Health Benefits:

❖ Quinoa provides protein and fiber, which help keep you feeling full and satisfied.

❖ Black beans are rich in fiber and plant-based protein, which help stabilize blood sugar levels and support digestive health.

Preparation Time: 15 minutes

LUNCH RECIPES

1: Quinoa and Black Bean Salad

Ingredients:

❖ 1 cup cooked quinoa
❖ 1 can (14 oz) black beans, rinsed and drained
❖ 1 cup diced bell peppers (any color)
❖ ½ cup diced red onion
❖ ½ cup corn kernels
❖ ¼ cup chopped fresh cilantro
❖ 2 tablespoons lime juice
❖ 2 tablespoons extra virgin olive oil
❖ 1 teaspoon cumin
❖ Salt and pepper to taste

Instructions:

- ❖ In a large bowl, combine cooked quinoa, black beans, diced bell peppers, diced red onion, corn kernels, and chopped fresh cilantro.
- ❖ In a separate small bowl, whisk together lime juice, extra virgin olive oil, cumin, salt, and pepper.
- ❖ Pour the dressing over the quinoa mixture and toss gently to combine all the ingredients.
- ❖ Adjust seasoning if needed.
- ❖ Serve chilled.

Health Benefits:

- ❖ Quinoa provides a complete protein source, essential for thyroid health.
- ❖ Black beans are rich in fiber, aiding digestion and promoting gut health.
- ❖ Bell peppers are high in vitamin C, supporting immune function.
- ❖ Olive oil provides healthy fats, which may reduce inflammation associated with Hashimoto's disease.
- ❖ Cumin may help improve digestion and reduce inflammation.

Preparation Time: 15 minutes

Ingredients:

- ❖ 1 cup cooked lentils
- ❖ 1 tablespoon olive oil
- ❖ 1 small onion, sliced
- ❖ 1 bell pepper, sliced
- ❖ 1 zucchini, sliced
- ❖ 1 cup sliced mushrooms
- ❖ 2 cloves garlic, minced
- ❖ 2 tablespoons low-sodium soy sauce
- ❖ 1 tablespoon rice vinegar
- ❖ 1 tablespoon chopped green onions (scallions)
- ❖ Salt and pepper to taste

Instructions:

- ❖ Heat olive oil in a large skillet or wok over medium heat.
- ❖ Add sliced onion, bell pepper, zucchini, and sliced mushrooms to the skillet. Stir-fry for 4-5 minutes or until the vegetables are tender-crisp.
- ❖ Add minced garlic and stir-fry for an additional minute.
- ❖ Add cooked lentils, soy sauce, rice vinegar, chopped green onions, salt, and pepper to the skillet. Stir-fry for another 2-3 minutes to combine the flavors.
- ❖ Remove from heat and serve hot.

Health Benefits:

- ❖ Lentils are rich in protein and fiber, promoting satiety and stabilizing blood sugar levels.
- ❖ Vegetables like bell peppers, zucchini, and mushrooms provide essential vitamins and minerals for overall health.
- ❖ Garlic may help reduce inflammation and support immune function.
- ❖ Soy sauce adds flavor without added salt, which is beneficial for managing blood pressure.

Preparation Time: 15 minutes

3: Chickpea Avocado Salad

Ingredients:

- ❖ 1 can (15 oz) chickpeas, rinsed and drained
- ❖ 1 ripe avocado, diced
- ❖ 1 cup cherry tomatoes, halved
- ❖ ½ cucumber, diced
- ❖ ¼ cup red onion, finely chopped
- ❖ 2 tablespoons chopped fresh parsley
- ❖ 1 tablespoon extra virgin olive oil
- ❖ 1 tablespoon lemon juice
- ❖ Salt and pepper to taste

Instructions:

- ❖ In a large bowl, combine chickpeas, diced avocado, cherry tomatoes, diced cucumber, red onion, and chopped parsley.
- ❖ Drizzle extra virgin olive oil and lemon juice over the salad.
- ❖ Season with salt and pepper to taste.
- ❖ Toss gently to combine all ingredients.
- ❖ Serve chilled or at room temperature.

Health Benefits:

- ❖ Chickpeas are rich in protein and fiber, promoting satiety and digestive health.
- ❖ Avocado provides healthy fats, potassium, and vitamins, supporting heart health and skin health.
- ❖ Tomatoes are high in antioxidants, including vitamin C and lycopene, which may reduce inflammation.
- ❖ Olive oil contains monounsaturated fats, which may help reduce the risk of heart disease.

Preparation Time: 10 minutes

4: Lentil Vegetable Soup

Ingredients:

- ❖ 1 tablespoon olive oil
- ❖ 1 onion, diced
- ❖ 2 carrots, diced

- ❖ 2 celery stalks, diced
- ❖ 2 cloves garlic, minced
- ❖ 1 cup dried green or brown lentils, rinsed
- ❖ 4 cups vegetable broth
- ❖ 1 can (14 oz) diced tomatoes
- ❖ 1 teaspoon dried thyme
- ❖ 1 teaspoon dried rosemary
- ❖ Salt and pepper to taste
- ❖ Fresh parsley for garnish (optional)

Instructions:

- ❖ In a large pot, heat olive oil over medium heat.
- ❖ Add diced onion, carrots, and celery. Cook until vegetables are softened, about 5 minutes.
- ❖ Add minced garlic and cook for another minute.
- ❖ Stir in dried lentils, vegetable broth, diced tomatoes (with their juices), dried thyme, and dried rosemary.
- ❖ Bring soup to a boil, then reduce heat to low. Cover and simmer for about 20-25 minutes, or until lentils are tender.
- ❖ Season with salt and pepper to taste.
- ❖ Serve hot, garnished with fresh parsley if desired.

Health Benefits:

- ❖ Lentils are an excellent source of plant-based protein, fiber, and essential nutrients, helping to stabilize blood sugar levels and promote satiety.
- ❖ Carrots and celery provide vitamins A and K, as well as antioxidants, supporting immune function and overall health.
- ❖ Garlic contains sulfur compounds with potential anti-inflammatory and immune-boosting properties.
- ❖ Tomatoes are rich in lycopene, an antioxidant that may reduce inflammation and protect against chronic diseases.

Preparation Time: 30 minutes

5: Sweet Potato and Black Bean Quesadillas

Ingredients:

- ❖ 2 medium sweet potatoes, peeled and diced
- ❖ 1 can (15 oz) black beans, rinsed and drained
- ❖ 1 teaspoon ground cumin
- ❖ 1 teaspoon chili powder
- ❖ ½ teaspoon garlic powder
- ❖ Salt and pepper to taste
- ❖ 4 large whole wheat or corn tortillas

❖ 1 cup shredded dairy-free cheese (such as vegan cheddar or mozzarella)

❖ Salsa, avocado, and cilantro for serving (optional)

Instructions:

❖ Place diced sweet potatoes in a microwave-safe bowl with a splash of water. Cover and microwave for 5-7 minutes, or until tender.

❖ In a separate bowl, mash the black beans with ground cumin, chili powder, garlic powder, salt, and pepper.

❖ Lay out tortillas and spread mashed black beans evenly on one half of each tortilla.

❖ Top with cooked sweet potatoes and shredded dairy-free cheese.

❖ Fold the tortillas in half to create quesadillas.

❖ Heat a large skillet over medium heat and cook each quesadilla for 2-3 minutes on each side, or until golden and crispy.

❖ Serve hot with salsa, avocado, and cilantro if desired.

Health Benefits:

❖ Sweet potatoes are rich in fiber, vitamins, and antioxidants, supporting gut health and immune function.

❖ Black beans are a good source of plant-based protein, fiber, and folate, promoting satiety and heart health.

❖ Whole wheat or corn tortillas provide complex carbohydrates for sustained energy levels.

❖ Dairy-free cheese offers a calcium-rich alternative for those avoiding dairy products.

Preparation Time: 20 minutes

6: Mediterranean Chickpea Salad

Ingredients:

❖ 2 cans (15 oz each) chickpeas, rinsed and drained

❖ 1 cucumber, diced

❖ 1 cup cherry tomatoes, halved

❖ ½ cup diced red onion

❖ ½ cup chopped fresh parsley

❖ ¼ cup sliced Kalamata olives

❖ 2 tablespoons extra virgin olive oil

❖ 2 tablespoons lemon juice

❖ 1 teaspoon dried oregano

❖ Salt and pepper to taste

❖ Crumbled feta cheese (optional)

Instructions:

❖ In a large bowl, combine chickpeas, diced cucumber, cherry tomatoes, diced red onion, chopped parsley, and sliced Kalamata olives.

❖ In a small bowl, whisk together extra virgin olive oil, lemon juice, dried oregano, salt, and pepper.

❖ Pour the dressing over the chickpea salad and toss gently to coat.

❖ Adjust seasoning if needed.

❖ Serve chilled, garnished with crumbled feta cheese if desired.

Health Benefits:

❖ Chickpeas provide plant-based protein and fiber, promoting satiety and digestive health.

❖ Cucumbers and tomatoes are hydrating and low in calories, while also providing vitamins and antioxidants.

❖ Olives and olive oil offer heart-healthy monounsaturated fats and antioxidants, reducing inflammation and supporting heart health.

❖ Parsley adds flavor and provides vitamins K and C, supporting bone health and immune function.

Preparation Time: 15 minutes

7: Roasted Vegetable Quinoa Bowl

Ingredients:

❖ 1 cup quinoa, rinsed

❖ 2 cups water or vegetable broth

- ❖ 1 medium sweet potato, peeled and diced
- ❖ 1 small eggplant, diced
- ❖ 1 red bell pepper, diced
- ❖ 1 zucchini, diced
- ❖ 1 tablespoon olive oil
- ❖ 1 teaspoon dried thyme
- ❖ 1 teaspoon dried rosemary
- ❖ Salt and pepper to taste
- ❖ 2 tablespoons tahini
- ❖ 1 tablespoon lemon juice
- ❖ 2 tablespoons chopped fresh parsley for garnish

Instructions:

- ❖ Preheat the oven to 400°F (200°C).
- ❖ In a saucepan, combine quinoa and water or vegetable broth. Bring to a boil, then reduce heat, cover, and simmer for 15-20 minutes, or until quinoa is cooked and water is absorbed.
- ❖ Meanwhile, spread diced sweet potato, eggplant, red bell pepper, and zucchini on a baking sheet. Drizzle with olive oil and sprinkle with dried thyme, dried rosemary, salt, and pepper. Toss to coat evenly.
- ❖ Roast the vegetables in the preheated oven for 20-25 minutes, or until tender and slightly caramelized.

- In a small bowl, whisk together tahini and lemon juice to make the dressing.
- To assemble the bowls, divide cooked quinoa among serving bowls. Top with roasted vegetables and drizzle with tahini dressing.
- Garnish with chopped fresh parsley before serving.

Health Benefits:

- Quinoa is a complete protein source, providing all essential amino acids necessary for overall health.
- Sweet potatoes, eggplant, bell peppers, and zucchini are rich in vitamins, minerals, and antioxidants, supporting immune function and reducing inflammation.
- Tahini is a good source of healthy fats and contains essential nutrients like calcium and iron.

Preparation Time: 35 minutes

8: Vegan Lentil Sloppy Joes

Ingredients:

- 1 cup dry green or brown lentils, rinsed
- 3 cups water or vegetable broth
- 1 tablespoon olive oil
- 1 onion, diced
- 2 cloves garlic, minced

- ❖ 1 red bell pepper, diced
- ❖ 1 carrot, grated
- ❖ 1 cup tomato sauce
- ❖ 2 tablespoons tomato paste
- ❖ 1 tablespoon maple syrup or coconut sugar
- ❖ 1 tablespoon apple cider vinegar
- ❖ 1 teaspoon smoked paprika
- ❖ 1 teaspoon chili powder
- ❖ Salt and pepper to taste
- ❖ 4 whole grain burger buns or lettuce leaves for serving

Instructions:

- ❖ In a saucepan, combine lentils and water or vegetable broth. Bring to a boil, then reduce heat, cover, and simmer for 20-25 minutes, or until lentils are tender but not mushy. Drain any excess liquid and set aside.
- ❖ In a large skillet, heat olive oil over medium heat. Add diced onion, minced garlic, diced red bell pepper, and grated carrot. Cook until vegetables are softened, about 5 minutes.
- ❖ Stir in cooked lentils, tomato sauce, tomato paste, maple syrup or coconut sugar, apple cider vinegar, smoked paprika, chili powder, salt, and pepper. Cook for an additional 5 minutes, stirring occasionally, until the mixture is heated through and flavors are well combined.

- ❖ To serve, spoon the lentil mixture onto whole grain burger buns or lettuce leaves for a low-carb option.

Health Benefits:

- ❖ Lentils are an excellent source of plant-based protein, fiber, and essential nutrients, supporting satiety and digestive health.
- ❖ Bell peppers and carrots are rich in antioxidants like vitamin C and beta-carotene, supporting immune function and reducing inflammation.
- ❖ Tomato sauce provides lycopene, a powerful antioxidant associated with reduced risk of chronic diseases like heart disease and cancer.

Preparation Time: 40 minutes

9: Mediterranean Chickpea Wrap

Ingredients:

- ❖ 1 can (15 oz) chickpeas, rinsed and drained
- ❖ 1/2 cucumber, diced
- ❖ 1/2 cup cherry tomatoes, halved
- ❖ 1/4 cup diced red onion
- ❖ 2 tablespoons chopped fresh parsley
- ❖ 2 tablespoons lemon juice
- ❖ 2 tablespoons extra virgin olive oil

- ❖ 1 teaspoon dried oregano
- ❖ Salt and pepper to taste
- ❖ 4 whole grain wraps or tortillas

Instructions:

- ❖ In a large bowl, combine chickpeas, diced cucumber, cherry tomatoes, diced red onion, and chopped parsley.
- ❖ In a small bowl, whisk together lemon juice, olive oil, dried oregano, salt, and pepper to make the dressing.
- ❖ Pour the dressing over the chickpea mixture and toss to coat evenly.
- ❖ Warm the whole grain wraps or tortillas according to package instructions.
- ❖ Divide the chickpea mixture evenly among the wraps or tortillas.
- ❖ Roll up the wraps tightly and slice in half.
- ❖ Serve immediately or wrap in foil for later.

Health Benefits:

- ❖ Chickpeas are rich in protein and fiber, promoting satiety and digestive health.
- ❖ Cucumbers and tomatoes provide hydration and essential vitamins and minerals.

* Olive oil offers heart-healthy monounsaturated fats and antioxidants, reducing inflammation and supporting heart health.
* Parsley adds flavor and contains vitamins K and C, supporting bone health and immune function.

Preparation Time: 15 minutes

10: Butternut Squash and Lentil Soup

Ingredients:

* 1 tablespoon olive oil
* 1 onion, diced
* 2 cloves garlic, minced
* 1 butternut squash, peeled, seeded, and diced
* 1 cup dried green or brown lentils, rinsed
* 4 cups vegetable broth
* 1 teaspoon ground cumin
* 1 teaspoon ground coriander
* Salt and pepper to taste
* Fresh parsley for garnish (optional)

Instructions:

* In a large pot, heat olive oil over medium heat.
* Add diced onion and minced garlic. Cook until softened, about 5 minutes.

- ❖ Add diced butternut squash and cook for another 5 minutes.
- ❖ Stir in dried lentils, vegetable broth, ground cumin, and ground coriander.
- ❖ Bring the soup to a boil, then reduce heat to low. Cover and simmer for 25-30 minutes, or until the lentils and squash are tender.
- ❖ Season with salt and pepper to taste.
- ❖ Garnish with fresh parsley before serving.

Health Benefits:

- ❖ Butternut squash is rich in vitamins A and C, as well as fiber, supporting immune function and digestive health.
- ❖ Lentils provide plant-based protein and fiber, promoting satiety and stabilizing blood sugar levels.
- ❖ Onions and garlic contain sulfur compounds with potential anti-inflammatory and immune-boosting properties.
- ❖ Vegetable broth adds flavor and hydration without added calories or fat.

Preparation Time: 40 minutes

DINNER RECIPES

1: Lentil and Vegetable Stew

Ingredients:

- ❖ 1 cup dried green or brown lentils, rinsed

- ❖ 4 cups vegetable broth
- ❖ 1 onion, chopped
- ❖ 2 carrots, diced
- ❖ 2 celery stalks, chopped
- ❖ 2 cloves garlic, minced
- ❖ 1 can (14 oz) diced tomatoes
- ❖ 2 cups chopped kale or spinach
- ❖ 1 teaspoon dried thyme
- ❖ 1 teaspoon dried rosemary
- ❖ Salt and pepper to taste
- ❖ 2 tablespoons olive oil

Instructions:

- ❖ In a large pot, heat olive oil over medium heat. Add chopped onion, carrots, and celery. Cook until vegetables are softened, about 5 minutes.
- ❖ Add minced garlic and cook for another minute.
- ❖ Stir in lentils, vegetable broth, diced tomatoes (with their juices), dried thyme, and dried rosemary. Bring to a boil.
- ❖ Reduce heat to low, cover, and simmer for 25-30 minutes or until lentils are tender.
- ❖ Add chopped kale or spinach and cook for an additional 5 minutes until wilted.
- ❖ Season with salt and pepper to taste.

❖ Serve hot, garnished with fresh herbs if desired.

Health Benefits:

❖ Lentils are rich in fiber and plant-based protein, which can help stabilize blood sugar levels and support gut health.

❖ The variety of vegetables provides essential vitamins, minerals, and antioxidants, which support immune function and reduce inflammation.

Preparation Time: 40 minutes

2: Roasted Vegetable Quinoa Bowl

Ingredients:

❖ 1 cup quinoa, rinsed

❖ 2 cups water or vegetable broth

❖ 1 sweet potato, peeled and diced

❖ 1 zucchini, sliced

❖ 1 red bell pepper, sliced

❖ 1 yellow bell pepper, sliced

❖ 1 red onion, sliced

❖ 2 tablespoons olive oil

❖ 1 teaspoon dried thyme

❖ 1 teaspoon smoked paprika

❖ Salt and pepper to taste

❖ Fresh parsley or cilantro for garnish (optional)

Instructions:

- ❖ Preheat the oven to 400°F (200°C). Line a baking sheet with parchment paper.
- ❖ In a bowl, toss diced sweet potato, sliced zucchini, sliced red bell pepper, sliced yellow bell pepper, and sliced red onion with olive oil, dried thyme, smoked paprika, salt, and pepper until evenly coated.
- ❖ Spread the vegetables in a single layer on the prepared baking sheet.
- ❖ Roast in the preheated oven for 25-30 minutes, stirring halfway through, until vegetables are tender and slightly caramelized.
- ❖ While the vegetables are roasting, prepare the quinoa. In a medium saucepan, bring water or vegetable broth to a boil. Stir in rinsed quinoa, reduce heat to low, cover, and simmer for 15-20 minutes or until quinoa is fluffy and water is absorbed.
- ❖ To serve, divide cooked quinoa among serving bowls and top with roasted vegetables.
- ❖ Garnish with fresh parsley or cilantro if desired.
- ❖ Serve hot or at room temperature.

Health Benefits:

- ❖ Quinoa is a complete protein source and rich in fiber, which can aid in digestion and help stabilize blood sugar levels.
- ❖ Roasted vegetables are packed with vitamins, minerals, and antioxidants, which support immune function and reduce inflammation.

Preparation Time: 45 minutes

3: Chickpea and Vegetable Stir-Fry

Ingredients:

- ❖ 1 can (14 oz) chickpeas, drained and rinsed
- ❖ 2 cups mixed vegetables (such as broccoli, bell peppers, carrots, snap peas)
- ❖ 1 onion, sliced
- ❖ 2 cloves garlic, minced
- ❖ 1 tablespoon ginger, grated
- ❖ 3 tablespoons low-sodium soy sauce or tamari
- ❖ 1 tablespoon maple syrup or coconut sugar
- ❖ 1 tablespoon rice vinegar
- ❖ 2 tablespoons sesame oil
- ❖ Cooked brown rice or quinoa, for serving
- ❖ Sesame seeds and chopped green onions, for garnish (optional)

Instructions:

- ❖ Heat sesame oil in a large skillet or wok over medium heat.
- ❖ Add sliced onion, minced garlic, and grated ginger. Stir-fry for 2-3 minutes until fragrant.
- ❖ Add mixed vegetables to the skillet and cook for 5-7 minutes until tender-crisp.
- ❖ Stir in chickpeas and cook for another 2-3 minutes.
- ❖ In a small bowl, whisk together soy sauce or tamari, maple syrup or coconut sugar, and rice vinegar. Pour the sauce over the vegetables and chickpeas, stirring to coat evenly.
- ❖ Cook for an additional 2-3 minutes until the sauce thickens slightly.
- ❖ Serve the stir-fry over cooked brown rice or quinoa.
- ❖ Garnish with sesame seeds and chopped green onions if desired.

Health Benefits:

- ❖ Chickpeas are a good source of plant-based protein and fiber, which can help stabilize blood sugar levels and promote satiety.
- ❖ The variety of colorful vegetables provides essential vitamins, minerals, and antioxidants, supporting overall health and immune function.

Preparation Time: 25 minutes

4: Stuffed Bell Peppers with Quinoa and Black Beans

Ingredients:

- ❖ 4 bell peppers (any color), halved and seeds removed
- ❖ 1 cup cooked quinoa
- ❖ 1 can (14 oz) black beans, rinsed and drained
- ❖ 1 cup diced tomatoes
- ❖ 1 cup corn kernels (fresh or frozen)
- ❖ 1 small onion, diced
- ❖ 2 cloves garlic, minced
- ❖ 1 teaspoon chili powder
- ❖ 1 teaspoon ground cumin
- ❖ Salt and pepper to taste
- ❖ Fresh cilantro, for garnish (optional)
- ❖ Lime wedges, for serving

Instructions:

- ❖ Preheat the oven to 375°F (190°C). Arrange bell pepper halves in a baking dish, cut side up.
- ❖ In a large skillet, heat olive oil over medium heat. Add diced onion and minced garlic, sautéing until softened, about 3-4 minutes.
- ❖ Add cooked quinoa, black beans, diced tomatoes, corn kernels, chili powder, ground cumin, salt, and pepper to the skillet. Stir to combine and cook for another 3-4 minutes.

- ❖ Spoon the quinoa and black bean mixture into the bell pepper halves, pressing down gently to fill.
- ❖ Cover the baking dish with foil and bake in the preheated oven for 25-30 minutes, until the peppers are tender.
- ❖ Remove foil and bake for an additional 5-10 minutes to lightly brown the tops.
- ❖ Garnish with fresh cilantro if desired and serve with lime wedges.

Health Benefits:

- ❖ Bell peppers are rich in vitamin C and antioxidants, supporting immune function and reducing inflammation.
- ❖ Quinoa and black beans provide plant-based protein, fiber, and essential nutrients, promoting stable blood sugar levels and satiety.

Preparation Time: 40 minutes

5: Mushroom and Lentil Shepherd's Pie

Ingredients:

- ❖ 1 cup green or brown lentils, rinsed
- ❖ 3 cups vegetable broth
- ❖ 2 tablespoons olive oil
- ❖ 1 onion, chopped
- ❖ 2 carrots, diced

- ❖ 2 celery stalks, diced

- ❖ 2 cloves garlic, minced

- ❖ 8 oz mushrooms, sliced

- ❖ 1 tablespoon tomato paste

- ❖ 1 teaspoon dried thyme

- ❖ 1 teaspoon dried rosemary

- ❖ Salt and pepper to taste

- ❖ 4 cups mashed sweet potatoes or mashed cauliflower

- ❖ Fresh parsley, for garnish (optional)

Instructions:

- ❖ Preheat the oven to 375°F (190°C). Grease a baking dish.

- ❖ In a medium saucepan, combine lentils and vegetable broth. Bring to a boil, then reduce heat and simmer for 20-25 minutes, or until lentils are tender and most of the liquid is absorbed.

- ❖ In a large skillet, heat olive oil over medium heat. Add chopped onion, carrots, celery, and minced garlic. Cook until vegetables are softened, about 5 minutes.

- ❖ Add sliced mushrooms to the skillet and cook for another 5 minutes, until mushrooms are browned.

- ❖ Stir in tomato paste, dried thyme, dried rosemary, salt, and pepper. Cook for 2 minutes.

- ❖ Add cooked lentils to the skillet and stir to combine.

- ❖ Transfer the lentil and vegetable mixture to the prepared baking dish.
- ❖ Spread mashed sweet potatoes or mashed cauliflower over the top.
- ❖ Bake in the preheated oven for 25-30 minutes, or until the filling is bubbly and the top is lightly golden.
- ❖ Garnish with fresh parsley if desired before serving.

Health Benefits:

- ❖ Lentils are a good source of plant-based protein and fiber, which can help stabilize blood sugar levels and promote satiety.
- ❖ Mushrooms are rich in antioxidants and may have immune-boosting properties, which can support overall health and well-being.

Preparation Time: 1 hour

6: Vegan Butternut Squash Risotto

Ingredients:

- ❖ 1 small butternut squash, peeled, seeded, and diced
- ❖ 2 tablespoons olive oil
- ❖ 1 onion, finely chopped
- ❖ 2 cloves garlic, minced
- ❖ 1 ½ cups Arborio rice

- ❖ 4 cups vegetable broth, warmed
- ❖ ½ cup dry white wine (optional)
- ❖ ½ cup nutritional yeast
- ❖ Salt and pepper to taste
- ❖ Fresh sage leaves, for garnish (optional)

Instructions:

- ❖ Preheat the oven to 400°F (200°C). Place diced butternut squash on a baking sheet, drizzle with 1 tablespoon of olive oil, and season with salt and pepper. Roast for 20-25 minutes, or until tender and lightly browned.
- ❖ In a large skillet or saucepan, heat remaining olive oil over medium heat. Add chopped onion and sauté until translucent, about 5 minutes. Add minced garlic and cook for another minute.
- ❖ Stir in Arborio rice and cook for 2-3 minutes, until rice is lightly toasted.
- ❖ Deglaze the pan with dry white wine, if using, and cook until the wine is absorbed.
- ❖ Gradually add warm vegetable broth, 1 cup at a time, stirring frequently and allowing the liquid to be absorbed before adding more.

- ❖ Once the rice is creamy and tender, stir in roasted butternut squash and nutritional yeast. Cook for another 2-3 minutes to heat through.
- ❖ Season with salt and pepper to taste.
- ❖ Serve hot, garnished with fresh sage leaves if desired.

Health Benefits:

- ❖ Butternut squash is rich in vitamins, minerals, and antioxidants, which support immune function and reduce inflammation.
- ❖ Arborio rice is a good source of complex carbohydrates, providing sustained energy and promoting satiety.

Preparation Time: 45 minutes

7: Cauliflower and Chickpea Curry

Ingredients:

- ❖ 1 head cauliflower, cut into florets
- ❖ 1 can (14 oz) chickpeas, drained and rinsed
- ❖ 1 onion, finely chopped
- ❖ 2 cloves garlic, minced
- ❖ 1-inch piece of ginger, grated
- ❖ 1 can (14 oz) diced tomatoes
- ❖ 1 can (14 oz) coconut milk
- ❖ 2 tablespoons curry powder

- ❖ 1 teaspoon ground turmeric
- ❖ 1 teaspoon ground cumin
- ❖ 1 teaspoon ground coriander
- ❖ Salt and pepper to taste
- ❖ Cooked brown rice or quinoa, for serving
- ❖ Fresh cilantro, for garnish (optional)

Instructions:

- ❖ In a large skillet or saucepan, heat olive oil over medium heat. Add chopped onion and cook until translucent, about 5 minutes.
- ❖ Add minced garlic and grated ginger, and cook for another minute.
- ❖ Stir in curry powder, ground turmeric, ground cumin, and ground coriander. Cook for 1-2 minutes until fragrant.
- ❖ Add diced tomatoes (with their juices) and coconut milk to the skillet. Stir to combine.
- ❖ Add cauliflower florets and chickpeas to the skillet. Bring the mixture to a simmer.
- ❖ Cover and cook for 15-20 minutes, or until the cauliflower is tender.
- ❖ Season with salt and pepper to taste.
- ❖ Serve the cauliflower and chickpea curry over cooked brown rice or quinoa.

❖ Garnish with fresh cilantro if desired.

Health Benefits:

❖ Cauliflower is a cruciferous vegetable rich in antioxidants and fiber, which can support immune function and reduce inflammation.
❖ Chickpeas are a good source of plant-based protein and fiber, promoting stable blood sugar levels and satiety.

Preparation Time: 40 minutes

8: Vegan Lentil Meatballs with Zucchini Noodles

Ingredients:

❖ 1 cup dried green or brown lentils, rinsed
❖ 3 cups vegetable broth
❖ 2 tablespoons ground flaxseeds
❖ 6 tablespoons water
❖ 1 onion, finely chopped
❖ 2 cloves garlic, minced
❖ 1 tablespoon tomato paste
❖ 1 teaspoon dried oregano
❖ 1 teaspoon dried basil
❖ Salt and pepper to taste
❖ 4 medium zucchinis, spiralized into noodles
❖ Olive oil for cooking

- ❖ Marinara sauce, for serving

- ❖ Fresh basil, for garnish (optional)

Instructions:

- ❖ In a medium saucepan, combine lentils and vegetable broth. Bring to a boil, then reduce heat and simmer for 20-25 minutes, or until lentils are tender and most of the liquid is absorbed.

- ❖ In a small bowl, mix ground flaxseeds and water. Let it sit for 5 minutes to thicken and form a gel-like consistency.

- ❖ In a large skillet, heat olive oil over medium heat. Add chopped onion and minced garlic, and sauté until softened, about 5 minutes.

- ❖ Stir in cooked lentils, flaxseed mixture, tomato paste, dried oregano, dried basil, salt, and pepper.

- ❖ Cook for another 5 minutes, until the mixture is heated through and well combined.

- ❖ Using your hands, shape the lentil mixture into meatballs.

- ❖ In the same skillet, heat more olive oil over medium heat. Add lentil meatballs and cook for 6-8 minutes, turning occasionally, until browned on all sides.

- ❖ Meanwhile, spiralize zucchinis into noodles.

- ❖ Serve lentil meatballs over zucchini noodles with marinara sauce.

❖ Garnish with fresh basil if desired.

Health Benefits:

❖ Lentils are a good source of plant-based protein and fiber, which can help stabilize blood sugar levels and promote satiety.

❖ Zucchini noodles are low in calories and carbohydrates, providing a lighter alternative to traditional pasta and supporting weight management.

Preparation Time: 45 minutes

9: Quinoa Stuffed Bell Peppers

Ingredients:

❖ 4 bell peppers (any color), halved and seeds removed

❖ 1 cup quinoa, rinsed

❖ 2 cups vegetable broth

❖ 1 can (14 oz) black beans, drained and rinsed

❖ 1 cup corn kernels (fresh or frozen)

❖ 1 onion, diced

❖ 2 cloves garlic, minced

❖ 1 teaspoon ground cumin

❖ 1 teaspoon chili powder

❖ Salt and pepper to taste

❖ 1 cup salsa

- ❖ 1 cup shredded vegan cheese (optional)
- ❖ Fresh cilantro, for garnish (optional)

Instructions:

- ❖ Preheat the oven to 375°F (190°C). Arrange bell pepper halves in a baking dish, cut side up.
- ❖ In a medium saucepan, bring vegetable broth to a boil. Stir in quinoa, reduce heat to low, cover, and simmer for 15-20 minutes or until quinoa is cooked and broth is absorbed.
- ❖ In a large skillet, heat olive oil over medium heat. Add diced onion and cook until translucent, about 5 minutes. Add minced garlic and cook for another minute.
- ❖ Stir in cooked quinoa, black beans, corn kernels, ground cumin, chili powder, salt, and pepper. Cook for 2-3 minutes until heated through.
- ❖ Spoon quinoa mixture into each bell pepper half until filled.
- ❖ Top each bell pepper half with salsa and shredded vegan cheese, if using.
- ❖ Cover the baking dish with foil and bake in the preheated oven for 25-30 minutes, or until bell peppers are tender.
- ❖ Garnish with fresh cilantro if desired before serving.

Health Benefits:

- ❖ Quinoa is a complete protein source and rich in fiber, which can help stabilize blood sugar levels and promote satiety.

❖ Black beans are packed with protein, fiber, and essential nutrients, supporting overall health and well-being.

Preparation Time: 45 minutes

10: Vegan Lentil Shepherd's Pie

Ingredients:

❖ 1 cup green or brown lentils, rinsed

❖ 3 cups vegetable broth

❖ 2 tablespoons olive oil

❖ 1 onion, chopped

❖ 2 carrots, diced

❖ 2 celery stalks, diced

❖ 2 cloves garlic, minced

❖ 8 oz mushrooms, sliced

❖ 1 tablespoon tomato paste

❖ 1 teaspoon dried thyme

❖ 1 teaspoon dried rosemary

❖ Salt and pepper to taste

❖ 4 cups mashed potatoes (made with plant-based milk and vegan butter)

❖ Fresh parsley, for garnish (optional)

Instructions:

❖ Preheat the oven to 375°F (190°C). Grease a baking dish.

- ❖ In a medium saucepan, combine lentils and vegetable broth. Bring to a boil, then reduce heat and simmer for 20-25 minutes, or until lentils are tender and most of the liquid is absorbed.
- ❖ In a large skillet, heat olive oil over medium heat. Add chopped onion, carrots, and celery. Cook until vegetables are softened, about 5 minutes.
- ❖ Add minced garlic and sliced mushrooms to the skillet. Cook for another 5 minutes until mushrooms are browned.
- ❖ Stir in tomato paste, dried thyme, dried rosemary, salt, and pepper. Cook for 2 minutes.
- ❖ Add cooked lentils to the skillet and stir to combine.
- ❖ Transfer the lentil and vegetable mixture to the prepared baking dish.
- ❖ Spread mashed potatoes over the top.
- ❖ Bake in the preheated oven for 25-30 minutes, or until the filling is bubbly and the top is lightly golden.
- ❖ Garnish with fresh parsley if desired before serving.

Health Benefits:

- ❖ Lentils are a good source of plant-based protein and fiber, which can help stabilize blood sugar levels and promote satiety.

❖ Mushrooms are rich in antioxidants and may have immune-boosting properties, which can support overall health and well-being.

Preparation Time: 1 hour

SNACK RECIPES

1: Avocado Toast with Hemp Seeds

Ingredients:

❖ 2 slices whole grain bread

❖ 1 ripe avocado

❖ 1 tablespoon hemp seeds

❖ Pinch of sea salt

❖ Pinch of red pepper flakes (optional)

❖ Fresh lemon juice (optional)

Instructions:

❖ Toast the slices of whole grain bread until golden brown.

❖ Mash the ripe avocado in a bowl until smooth and creamy.

❖ Spread the mashed avocado evenly onto the toasted bread slices.

❖ Sprinkle hemp seeds over the avocado toast.

❖ Add a pinch of sea salt and red pepper flakes if desired.

❖ Optionally, drizzle fresh lemon juice over the top.

❖ Serve immediately and enjoy!

Health Benefits:

- ❖ Avocado is rich in healthy fats, fiber, and potassium, which supports heart health and may help reduce inflammation.
- ❖ Hemp seeds are a good source of plant-based protein, omega-3 fatty acids, and minerals like magnesium and iron, which contribute to overall well-being and may support thyroid function.

Preparation Time: 10 minutes

2: Berry Chia Pudding

Ingredients:

- ❖ 1/4 cup chia seeds
- ❖ 1 cup unsweetened almond milk
- ❖ 1/2 teaspoon vanilla extract
- ❖ 1 tablespoon maple syrup or honey (optional)
- ❖ 1/2 cup mixed berries (strawberries, blueberries, raspberries)
- ❖ 2 tablespoons chopped nuts (almonds, walnuts, or pecans)

Instructions:

- ❖ In a bowl, mix chia seeds, almond milk, vanilla extract, and maple syrup or honey (if using).
- ❖ Stir well to combine,
- ❖ then let it sit for 10 minutes to allow the chia seeds to swell and thicken the mixture.

* Stir the mixture again to break up any clumps.
* Cover the bowl and refrigerate for at least 2 hours or overnight.
* When ready to serve, layer the chia pudding and mixed berries in glasses or bowls.
* Top with chopped nuts for added crunch and nutrition.
* Serve chilled and enjoy!

Health Benefits:

* Chia seeds are rich in omega-3 fatty acids, fiber, and antioxidants, which may help reduce inflammation and support heart health.
* Berries are packed with vitamins, minerals, and antioxidants, known for their anti-inflammatory properties and potential to support immune function.

Preparation Time: 15 minutes (plus chilling time)

3: Hummus and Veggie Platter

Ingredients:

* 1 cup homemade or store-bought hummus
* Assorted vegetables for dipping (carrot sticks, cucumber slices, bell pepper strips, cherry tomatoes, etc.)

Instructions:

* ❖ Arrange the hummus in the center of a serving platter.
* ❖ Surround the hummus with an assortment of colorful vegetables for dipping.
* ❖ Serve immediately and enjoy the crunchy, flavorful combination of veggies and hummus.

Health Benefits:

* ❖ Hummus is made from chickpeas, which are rich in protein, fiber, and essential nutrients like iron and folate. It provides sustained energy and supports digestive health.
* ❖ Assorted vegetables offer a variety of vitamins, minerals, and antioxidants that promote overall health and reduce inflammation, supporting optimal thyroid function.

Preparation Time: 10 minutes

4: Almond Butter Banana Bites

Ingredients:

* ❖ 2 ripe bananas
* ❖ 2 tablespoons almond butter
* ❖ 2 tablespoons unsweetened shredded coconut
* ❖ 2 tablespoons chopped almonds or walnuts

Instructions:

- ❖ Peel the bananas and cut them into thick slices.
- ❖ Spread a thin layer of almond butter on each banana slice.
- ❖ Sprinkle shredded coconut and chopped almonds or walnuts on top of the almond butter.
- ❖ Place the banana bites on a plate or tray and freeze for 30 minutes to firm up.
- ❖ Remove from the freezer and serve chilled.

Health Benefits:

- ❖ Bananas are a great source of potassium and fiber, which can help regulate blood sugar levels and support heart health.
- ❖ Almond butter is rich in healthy fats, protein, and magnesium, providing sustained energy and promoting satiety. It also contains vitamin E, an antioxidant that supports immune function.

Preparation Time: 10 minutes (plus chilling time)

5: Green Smoothie

Ingredients:

- ❖ 1 ripe banana
- ❖ 1 cup fresh spinach leaves
- ❖ 1/2 cup frozen pineapple chunks
- ❖ 1/2 cup unsweetened almond milk

- ❖ 1 tablespoon chia seeds
- ❖ 1 teaspoon grated ginger (optional)
- ❖ Ice cubes (optional)

Instructions:

- ❖ In a blender, combine the banana, spinach leaves, frozen pineapple chunks, almond milk, chia seeds, and grated ginger.
- ❖ Blend until smooth and creamy.
- ❖ Add ice cubes if a colder and thicker consistency is desired, then blend again.
- ❖ Pour into glasses and serve immediately.

Health Benefits:

- ❖ Spinach is a nutrient powerhouse, rich in vitamins A, C, and K, as well as iron, folate, and magnesium. It supports immune function and helps reduce inflammation.
- ❖ Pineapple contains bromelain, an enzyme known for its anti-inflammatory properties. It also provides vitamin C and manganese, which support overall health and immune function.

Preparation Time: 5 minutes

6: Roasted Chickpeas

Ingredients:

- ❖ 1 can (15 oz) chickpeas, drained, rinsed, and patted dry
- ❖ 1 tablespoon olive oil
- ❖ 1 teaspoon ground cumin
- ❖ 1/2 teaspoon smoked paprika
- ❖ 1/2 teaspoon garlic powder
- ❖ 1/4 teaspoon cayenne pepper (optional)
- ❖ Salt to taste

Instructions:

- ❖ Preheat the oven to 400°F (200°C) and line a baking sheet with parchment paper.
- ❖ In a bowl, toss the chickpeas with olive oil, ground cumin, smoked paprika, garlic powder, cayenne pepper (if using), and salt until evenly coated.
- ❖ Spread the seasoned chickpeas in a single layer on the prepared baking sheet.
- ❖ Roast in the preheated oven for 20-25 minutes, shaking the pan halfway through, until the chickpeas are crispy and golden brown.
- ❖ Remove from the oven and let cool slightly before serving.

Health Benefits:

❖ Chickpeas are an excellent source of plant-based protein, fiber, and various vitamins and minerals, including folate, iron, and manganese. They support digestive health, regulate blood sugar levels, and promote satiety.

Preparation Time: 30 minutes

7: Cucumber Slices with Tahini Dip

Ingredients:

❖ 1 large cucumber, sliced
❖ 2 tablespoons tahini
❖ 1 tablespoon lemon juice
❖ 1 clove garlic, minced
❖ Pinch of salt
❖ Pinch of paprika (optional)
❖ Fresh parsley, chopped (for garnish)

Instructions:

❖ In a small bowl, whisk together tahini, lemon juice, minced garlic, salt, and paprika (if using) until smooth.
❖ Arrange the cucumber slices on a serving plate.
❖ Drizzle the tahini dip over the cucumber slices.
❖ Garnish with chopped fresh parsley.
❖ Serve immediately and enjoy the refreshing flavors.

Health Benefits:

- ❖ Cucumbers are low in calories and high in water content, making them hydrating and refreshing. They also provide vitamins K and C, as well as antioxidants that support overall health.
- ❖ Tahini is made from ground sesame seeds and is rich in healthy fats, protein, and minerals like calcium and iron. It provides sustained energy and promotes heart health.

Preparation Time: 10 minutes

8: Quinoa and Veggie Stuffed Bell Peppers

Ingredients:

- ❖ 2 large bell peppers, halved and seeds removed
- ❖ 1 cup cooked quinoa
- ❖ 1/2 cup black beans, drained and rinsed
- ❖ 1/2 cup corn kernels (fresh, canned, or frozen)
- ❖ 1/2 cup diced tomatoes
- ❖ 1/4 cup diced red onion
- ❖ 1/4 cup chopped fresh cilantro
- ❖ 1 teaspoon ground cumin
- ❖ 1/2 teaspoon chili powder
- ❖ Salt and pepper to taste

Instructions:

- ❖ Preheat the oven to 375°F (190°C) and line a baking dish with parchment paper.
- ❖ In a large bowl, combine cooked quinoa, black beans, corn kernels, diced tomatoes, diced red onion, chopped fresh cilantro, ground cumin, chili powder, salt, and pepper.
- ❖ Spoon the quinoa mixture into the halved bell peppers, pressing down gently to pack the filling.
- ❖ Place the stuffed bell peppers in the prepared baking dish.
- ❖ Cover the dish with aluminum foil and bake in the preheated oven for 25-30 minutes, or until the peppers are tender.
- ❖ Remove from the oven and let cool slightly before serving.

Health Benefits:

- ❖ Bell peppers are rich in vitamins A and C, as well as antioxidants that support immune function and reduce inflammation.
- ❖ Quinoa is a complete protein source, providing all nine essential amino acids, along with fiber and various vitamins and minerals. It supports muscle repair, digestion, and overall health.

Preparation Time: 45 minutes

9: Edamame Hummus

Ingredients:

* 1 cup shelled edamame (fresh or frozen)
* 2 tablespoons tahini
* 2 tablespoons lemon juice
* 1 clove garlic, minced
* 2 tablespoons olive oil
* Salt and pepper to taste
* Pinch of paprika (for garnish)

Instructions:

* If using frozen edamame, cook according to package instructions until tender. If using fresh edamame, steam or boil until tender.
* In a food processor, combine the cooked edamame, tahini, lemon juice, minced garlic, olive oil, salt, and pepper.
* Blend until smooth, scraping down the sides as needed to ensure all ingredients are well combined.
* Transfer the edamame hummus to a serving bowl.
* Drizzle with a little extra olive oil and sprinkle with paprika for garnish.
* Serve with sliced vegetables or whole grain crackers for dipping.

Health Benefits:

- ❖ Edamame is a good source of plant-based protein, fiber, and various vitamins and minerals, including folate and vitamin K. It supports muscle repair, bone health, and overall well-being.
- ❖ Tahini provides healthy fats, protein, and minerals like calcium and iron, supporting heart health and energy production.

Preparation Time: 15 minutes

10: Baked Sweet Potato Chips

Ingredients:

- ❖ 2 medium sweet potatoes, scrubbed and thinly sliced
- ❖ 2 tablespoons olive oil
- ❖ 1 teaspoon smoked paprika
- ❖ 1/2 teaspoon garlic powder
- ❖ 1/2 teaspoon sea salt
- ❖ Fresh parsley, chopped (for garnish)

Instructions:

- ❖ Preheat the oven to 375°F (190°C) and line two baking sheets with parchment paper.

* In a large bowl, toss the thinly sliced sweet potatoes with olive oil, smoked paprika, garlic powder, and sea salt until evenly coated.
* Arrange the sweet potato slices in a single layer on the prepared baking sheets, making sure they don't overlap.
* Bake in the preheated oven for 15-20 minutes, flipping the chips halfway through, until golden and crispy.
* Remove from the oven and let cool slightly before serving.
* Sprinkle with chopped fresh parsley for garnish, if desired.

Health Benefits:

* Sweet potatoes are rich in vitamins A and C, as well as fiber and antioxidants that support immune function and reduce inflammation.
* Olive oil provides healthy monounsaturated fats and antioxidants, promoting heart health and reducing the risk of chronic disease.

Preparation Time: 30 minutes

Tips for Success on a Plant-Based Diet for Hashimoto's Disease/ Conclusion

Transitioning to a plant-based diet can be a beneficial step in managing

Hashimoto's disease, but it may also come with challenges. Here are some tips to help you successfully navigate a plant-based diet while effectively managing Hashimoto's disease:

Educate Yourself: Take the time to learn about Hashimoto's disease, its symptoms, and how diet can impact thyroid health. Understanding the relationship between food and autoimmune conditions can empower you to make informed dietary choices.

Consult with a Healthcare Professional: Before making any significant dietary changes, consult with a healthcare professional, such as a registered dietitian or endocrinologist, who can provide personalized guidance and support based on your individual health needs and medical history.

Focus on Nutrient Density: Emphasize whole, nutrient-dense plant foods in your diet, including fruits, vegetables, legumes, whole grains, nuts, and seeds. These foods are rich in vitamins, minerals, antioxidants, and fiber, which are essential for supporting immune function, reducing inflammation, and promoting overall health.

Ensure Adequate Protein Intake: Protein is important for muscle repair, immune function, and hormone production. Include plant-based sources of protein in your meals, such as beans, lentils, tofu, tempeh, edamame, quinoa, and nuts, to meet your daily protein needs.

Prioritize Omega-3 Fatty Acids: Omega-3 fatty acids have anti-inflammatory properties and may help reduce inflammation associated with autoimmune conditions like Hashimoto's disease. Include plant-based sources of omega-3s in your diet, such as flaxseeds, chia seeds, hemp seeds, walnuts, and algae-based supplements.

Monitor Iodine Intake: While iodine is essential for thyroid function, excessive iodine intake can exacerbate thyroid inflammation in individuals with Hashimoto's disease. Be mindful of your iodine intake and avoid consuming excessive amounts of iodine-rich foods, such as seaweed and iodized salt.

Stay Hydrated: Adequate hydration is important for supporting overall health and optimizing metabolic function. Drink plenty of water throughout the day and limit consumption of sugary beverages and caffeinated drinks, which can interfere with thyroid function.

Experiment with Recipes: Explore new plant-based recipes and experiment with different ingredients, flavors, and cooking methods to keep your meals interesting and enjoyable. Get creative in the kitchen and discover delicious plant-based alternatives to your favorite dishes.

Plan Ahead: Take time to plan your meals and snacks in advance to ensure that you have nutritious plant-based options readily available. Batch cooking and meal prepping can help save time and make healthy eating more convenient.

Listen to Your Body: Pay attention to how different foods make you feel and listen to your body's cues. Notice any changes in energy levels, digestion, or symptoms of Hashimoto's disease, and adjust your diet accordingly.